CHAIR YOGA FOR MEN OVER 50

A Comprehensive Strategies for Enhanced Mobility, Improved Strength, and Deepened Flexibility Without Standing

Carlos McDaniel

Table Of Content

Introduction — 4

Welcome and Overview — 7

Benefits of Chair Yoga for Men Over 50 — 10

Understanding Your Body at 50+ — 13

How to Use This Guide — 16

Getting Started — 19

Setting Up Your Space — 19

Choosing the Right Chair — 22

Safety Tips and Modifications — 25

Warm-Up and Cool-Down: Why They Matter — 28

Fundamental Chair Yoga Poses — 31

Seated Mountain Pose — 31

Chair Cat-Cow Stretch — 35

Seated Forward Bend — 38

Chair Extended Side Angle — 41

Seated Spinal Twist — 45

Seated Warrior Poses — 49

Strength Building with Chair Yoga — 53

Seated Chair Sun Salutations — 53

Chair Plank Variations — 57

Improving Flexibility — 64

Gentle Seated Stretches — 64

Shoulder and Neck Release   67

Enhancing Balance and Stability   **73**

Chair-Assisted Standing Poses   73

Relaxation and Stress Reduction   **83**

Guided Breathing Exercises   83

Seated Meditation Techniques   87

The Role of Mindfulness in Stress Reduction   89

Yoga Sequences for Specific Needs   **93**

Yoga for Back Pain Relief   93

Lifestyle and Wellness   **95**

Incorporating Yoga Principles into Daily Life   95

Nutrition Tips for Men Over 50   98

The Importance of Hydration   101

Conclusion   **105**

BONUS INSIDE TO THANK READER FOR
PURCHASING THIS BOOK

Inside this book after the conclusion, you will have access to somatic workout tracker journal and the audio version of this book.

Introduction

Richard lived in Maplewood, a quaint town nestled among the vibrant autumn trees. Richard, 55, had led an adventurous life, but recent years had left him feeling physically limited. His joints ached, his flexibility had waned, and his enthusiasm for outdoor activities seemed like a distant memory. Richard's doctor had mentioned yoga as a possible way to regain some of his mobility and vitality, but the thought of twisting into complex poses was daunting. That was until he came across a guide titled "Chair Yoga for Men Over 50."

The guide promised a transformative journey that did not require reaching the floor or standing for extended periods of time. It was designed specifically for men like Richard who wanted to reclaim their physical independence but needed a gentle push in the right direction. Richard decided to give it a shot, despite his initial reservations.

The first chapter greeted him with empathy and compassion, recognizing the difficulties that men over 50 face when starting a new physical routine. It mentioned the advantages of chair yoga, such as increased flexibility, stronger muscles, better balance, and lower stress. These weren't empty promises; they were backed up by testimonials from men who had traveled the same path Richard was about to embark on.

As Richard progressed through the chapters, he realized that chair yoga was more than just physical wellness; it was a comprehensive approach to living a balanced life. The guide gave clear, step-by-step instructions for each pose, complete with illustrations. There were modifications for every level of mobility, so Richard would never feel left behind. The section on safety tips and modifications was especially useful, as it taught him how to listen to his body and avoid injury.

The strength-building chapter surprised him by demonstrating that a chair could be an effective tool for building muscle without putting him at risk of strain. The flexibility section was a revelation, allowing him to gradually regain some of the range of motion he thought he'd lost permanently.

But it was the chapters on balance and stability that really changed Richard's perspective. He discovered a new sense of grounding through chair-assisted standing poses, as well as a way to stand strong in the face of life's uncertainties. The relaxation and stress reduction section taught him breathing exercises and meditation techniques that helped him maintain a sense of calm and mindfulness in his daily life.

As the weeks and months passed, Richard found himself not only practicing chair yoga, but also living it. He began to apply the principles of balance, flexibility, and strength to all aspects of his life, from his approach to work to his interactions with family and friends.

The guidebook, "Chair Yoga for Men Over 50," promised a transformative journey, and it delivered. Richard was more than just a participant; he had become a symbol of the power of starting where you are and working with what you have. He recommended the guide to his friends, eager to pass on the gift that had given him so much.

In the end, Richard's story was more than just chair yoga. It was about finding a path to wellness that respected his body's limitations while pushing him to become stronger, more flexible, and more balanced, both physically and mentally. Richard would advise anyone who is at a crossroads between wanting to improve their health and not knowing where to begin, "Buy this guide." It's not just about practicing yoga; it's about living a life in which age does not limit your abilities."

Welcome and Overview

Chair yoga offers a unique and transformative opportunity, particularly for men over the age of 50. This practice, which uses a chair to modify traditional yoga poses for accessibility and safety, provides a pathway to better health and well-being without the intimidation or risk associated with more traditional forms of exercise. It's designed to meet you where you're at in your fitness journey, recognizing the changes our bodies go through as we age and providing a supportive path to maintaining and improving physical and mental health.

For many men in this demographic, the prospect of starting a new physical activity is intimidating. Concerns about flexibility, injury, or simply knowing where to start are common. Chair yoga directly addresses these concerns by providing a low-impact, highly adaptable form of exercise that can significantly improve flexibility, strength, balance, and stress levels. It's a method that acknowledges the individual's current physical condition while gently encouraging progress and growth.

One of the most appealing aspects of chair yoga is its convenience. The use of a chair as a prop facilitates yoga poses and reduces strain on muscles and joints. This modification is critical for those who are dealing with chronic conditions or the natural decrease in flexibility and muscle mass that occurs with age. It enables practitioners to engage in a physical practice that respects their bodies' needs and limitations, bringing the benefits of yoga to a wider audience.

Chair yoga promotes a holistic approach to wellness. Aside from the physical benefits, it includes breathing exercises and meditation, which promote mental and emotional health. These techniques can help manage stress, improve focus, and promote a sense of calm and well-being. For men over 50, who frequently face the pressures of career, family responsibilities, and societal expectations, chair yoga's mental health benefits can be just as significant as the physical ones.

Chair yoga can help men over 50 overcome joint stiffness, muscle weakness, and balance issues. Regular practice can improve mobility and reduce the risk of falls, which is a growing concern as people age. Furthermore, the strength-building benefits of chair yoga can help counteract muscle loss, improving overall health and functionality.

Another significant advantage of chair yoga is the sense of community it can create. Joining a class or practicing with a group, even virtually, provides social interaction and support, which can be beneficial to mental health. This sense of belonging and shared experience can be extremely motivating, making it easier to stick with regular practice. For men who are retired or in transition in their careers, the community aspect of chair yoga provides a valuable opportunity to connect with others in a meaningful way.

Finally, chair yoga is an effective tool for men over the age of 50 who want to improve their overall well-being. It recognizes the unique challenges and opportunities that come with aging, providing an approach to better physical and mental health that is both accessible and enjoyable. Whether you want to improve your flexibility, strength, balance, or simply find a new way to relax and relieve stress, chair yoga has something for you. It's an invitation to discover the possibilities for growth and well-being, regardless of age or fitness level.

Benefits of Chair Yoga for Men Over 50

Chair yoga is a gentle yet effective form of exercise designed to meet the specific physical needs and challenges that men over 50 frequently face. This type of yoga uses a chair as a prop to perform various poses and stretches, making it more accessible to people with mobility issues, chronic conditions, or anyone who finds traditional yoga intimidating. Chair yoga, with regular practice, improves flexibility, which is essential for maintaining a healthy range of motion in the joints. As men age, their muscles and joints stiffen, resulting in decreased mobility and a higher risk of injury. Chair yoga addresses these concerns by gradually stretching and lengthening the muscles, increasing flexibility and making daily activities more manageable and comfortable.

Chair yoga not only improves flexibility, but it also significantly increases muscle strength. Strength training is essential for men over 50 because it helps to counteract the natural loss of muscle mass and bone density that occurs with age. Chair yoga can strengthen core, arm, leg, and back muscles by using the body's weight and resistance from various poses. This increased muscle strength improves joint health, lowers the risk of falling, and encourages a more active and independent lifestyle.

Balance is another area where chair yoga is extremely beneficial. Balance deteriorates with age, increasing the risk of falls and associated injuries. Chair yoga improves proprioception by focusing on movements and poses that engage the core and improve stability. This improved sense of balance can make navigating daily life safer and help to prevent falls, which are a common concern among men of this age.

Chair yoga has significant mental health benefits, including stress reduction and mental clarity. The practice includes breathing exercises and meditation, which can help reduce stress, anxiety, and promote overall well-being. The calming effect of chair yoga provides a much-needed mental respite for men over 50 who may be going through various life transitions or have health concerns. It also helps with emotional balance and offers a peaceful break from the stresses of everyday life.

Chair yoga can also improve cardiovascular health. Gentle yoga exercises can help lower blood pressure and improve circulation, both of which are important for cardiovascular health. These advantages are especially important for men over 50, who may be at a higher risk of heart disease and stroke. Chair yoga promotes relaxation and improves physical health, which helps to maintain a healthy heart and lowers the risk of cardiovascular disease.

Another benefit of chair yoga for men over 50 is its ability to improve sleep quality. Deep breathing and mindfulness, two relaxation techniques taught in chair yoga, can help improve sleep patterns. Better sleep boosts energy, mood, and overall health. This is especially beneficial for older men who may have sleep disturbances, allowing them to get deeper, more restorative sleep.

Finally, chair yoga encourages social interaction and a sense of community. Joining a chair yoga class allows you to meet people with similar interests and life experiences. This social interaction can be extremely beneficial to men over the age of 50, providing emotional support and alleviating feelings of isolation or loneliness. Through shared experiences in class, participants can build friendships and enjoy a sense of belonging, improving their overall quality of life.

Understanding Your Body at 50+

Men's bodies endure substantial modifications when they enter their fifties, which can have an influence on their physical health and general wellbeing. This stage of life is generally associated with a loss of muscular mass and flexibility, a slower metabolism, and an increased risk of chronic illnesses such as arthritis, hypertension, and heart disease. These changes can make traditional kinds of exercise more difficult, prompting many people to look for new ways to keep active and healthy. Chair yoga emerges as a particularly accessible type of exercise for men over 50, providing a gentle yet effective technique to address the physical changes associated with aging.

Chair yoga is created with the assumption that mobility and flexibility may be impaired in this age range. Using a chair as a prop gives stability and support, allowing practitioners to complete yoga postures with less strain on their joints and muscles. This versatility makes it a perfect workout for anyone suffering from joint discomfort or stiffness, as it allows them to gently stretch and strengthen their bodies without risking damage. The concentration on regulated movements and breathing also helps to improve balance and proprioception, which can be especially useful when these abilities deteriorate with age.

One of the primary benefits of chair yoga for men over 50 is its emphasis on flexibility. Muscles and joints might become less flexible as we age, resulting in a reduced range of motion and greater pain during regular tasks. Chair yoga gently exercises the body through a series of positions that stretch and lengthen the muscles, counteracting the effects of aging and sedentary lives. This enhanced flexibility can lead to better performance in other physical pursuits and fewer accidents.

Strength training is another important component of chair yoga, since it addresses the muscle mass loss that is frequent in older persons. The practice consists of postures and motions that use the body's weight or the chair's resistance to strengthen muscles, notably in the core, arms, and legs. This strengthening can assist men over 50 maintain metabolic health, promote bone density, and provide the strength they need for daily chores, resulting in an improved quality of life and increased independence.

Chair yoga also tackles the balance and stability issues that accompany aging. Practitioners can improve their sense of balance by doing concentrated postures and exercises that develop body awareness, lowering their chance of falling, which is a significant issue among older persons. The practice promotes awareness and attention, which aids in the development of balance and coordination abilities required for safe movement and participation in a variety of activities.

Furthermore, chair yoga promotes stress reduction and mental well-being. The contemplative features of yoga, paired with deep breathing techniques, encourage relaxation and mental clarity. Stress management is critical for men over 50 since persistent stress can worsen physical problems and have an influence on mental wellness. Chair yoga, with regular practice, can provide a sense of calm and resilience, improve sleep patterns, and alleviate symptoms of anxiety and sadness.

In essence, chair yoga provides a complete approach to tackling the physical and emotional issues that men confront as they enter their fifties and beyond. It offers a safe, adaptive, and effective strategy to maintain and enhance health while meeting the specific demands of this group. Men over 50 who practice chair yoga can benefit from greater flexibility, strength, balance, and mental well-being, which will help them live a more active, healthy, and meaningful lifestyle as they age.

How to Use This Guide

Embarking on a journey with chair yoga, particularly for men over 50, necessitates knowing that this guide is more than simply a collection of postures; it is a road to improved well-being, built with this demographic's specific requirements in mind. The technique is key to successfully utilize this tutorial. Begin by setting realistic expectations for yourself, acknowledging that growth in yoga, like life, is a series of ebbs and flows. It is critical to practice patience and allow oneself the freedom to grow at your own speed, noticing and applauding each tiny achievement along the road.

The guide is designed to progressively expose you to the foundations of chair yoga, ensuring that a strong foundation is established before moving on to more difficult sequences. This slow growth is critical to avoiding damage and increasing confidence. It recommends starting with the portions that cover fundamental postures and breathing methods. These first steps are critical because they create the framework for your practice, teaching you how to breathe efficiently and maintain perfect alignment, both of which are necessary for receiving the full benefits of yoga and avoiding injury.

As you get more acquainted with the fundamentals, the book invites you to explore chapters on strength, flexibility, and balance. It's designed for you to explore at your leisure, giving you the opportunity to concentrate on areas that correspond to your particular health objectives or treat specific physical difficulties. Whether it's strengthening joint health, increasing stability, or cultivating mental peace, each part includes a range of activities to ensure there's something for everyone. By choosing sequences that align with your goals, you can build a personalized yoga practice that is both pleasurable and useful.

Incorporating frequent practice into your everyday routine is another critical component of using this program effectively. Consistency is more important than the length of each session, so even a few minutes of practice every day can result in considerable gains over time. The approach is intended to be adaptable, allowing you to include yoga into your schedule, whether it's a morning routine to boost your energy or an evening practice to encourage relaxation and peaceful sleep.

The guide also highlights the value of mindfulness and the use of yoga concepts in daily life. Chair yoga is more than simply physical movement; it is about building a mindful attitude to daily tasks, fostering a stronger bond between mind and body. This comprehensive approach reduces stress and improves general quality of life, making yoga an effective tool for negotiating the challenges of this time of life.

To develop your practice, the book recommends contemplation and writing as a tool to assess progress and create goals. This introspective practice may be quite useful, providing insights into how yoga affects not just your physical health, but also your mental and emotional well-being. By documenting your experiences, you may track the transformational journey and change your practice as required to correspond with your changing objectives and requirements.

Finally, the handbook is intended to be a live resource, one to which you may return for inspiration, guidance, and support. As your requirements evolve, you may find other portions of the book more relevant, fostering a dynamic connection with your practice. This versatility is what makes chair yoga a durable friend for men over 50, providing a means to age gracefully, preserve independence, and enjoy a higher quality of life thanks to yoga's numerous advantages. This book is your beginning point, but ultimately, your practice is a personal journey that develops differently for each person who begins on it.

Getting Started

Setting Up Your Space

Creating a proper atmosphere for chair yoga, particularly for men over 50, begins with finding a quiet, comfortable location with few interruptions. This space does not have to be big, but it should be large enough to fit a chair and allow for unrestricted mobility of the arms and legs without colliding with any obstacles. Ideally, this location will become a sanctuary, allowing people to focus on movement, breathing, and relaxation without being distracted by the outside world. Natural light may improve mood and energy levels during practice, but if it isn't accessible, making sure the area is well-lit with soft, soothing artificial light can also help to create a tranquil environment.

Choosing the correct chair is essential for practicing chair yoga. The chair should be solid and without wheels to ensure stability during workouts. It should also feature a level seat that allows the feet to rest comfortably on the ground while sitting, with the knees bent at a proper angle. Armrests are optional; some people find them useful for particular positions, while others prefer a chair without them for more range of movement. During practice, the chair becomes an extension of the body, thus choosing it must consider not just comfort but also the ability to sustain weight and movement without shifting or tipping.

Another important factor to consider is the surface on which the chair is situated. A level, nonslip surface is essential for keeping the chair from moving abruptly. When practicing on a smooth floor, a non-slip yoga mat under the chair can enhance stability. For those on carpet, ensuring that the chair is firm and does not sink too far into the pile is critical, since this might compromise posture and balance.

Personalizing the room may greatly improve the chair yoga experience. Plants, photos, or simple decorations may be used to create an atmosphere of serenity and quiet. The goal is to create a setting that fosters a sense of well-being and motivates people to practice consistently. A small table or shelf within reach can be beneficial for storing water, a towel, or any other objects that may be required throughout the session, allowing for a smooth and continuous practice.

Sound is essential in creating an environment conducive to chair yoga. Incorporating moderate, peaceful music or natural sounds can assist to create an immersive experience that promotes deeper relaxation and attention. Alternatively, some people may choose to practice in quiet, which allows them to focus solely on their breathing and movement. The objective is to experiment with what best helps you stay focused and in a meditative state during your practice.

Temperature and ventilation should not be disregarded. To avoid distractions from practice or muscular tense-ups, keep the space at a pleasant temperature that is neither too hot nor too chilly. Good ventilation is also necessary to maintain a fresh supply of air, which helps to keep the mind alert and concentrated. If the room is stuffy, opening a window before starting might assist circulate air without causing a draft.

Finally, the issue of privacy is crucial. Chair yoga is a personal journey, and feeling safe in one's own space may have a tremendous impact on one's willingness to explore and actively participate in the practice. If you live with others, expressing the value of this time and confirming that there will be no interruptions can help you maintain a consistent and respected pattern. This designated time and place for chair yoga not only contributes to physical well-being but also to mental and emotional health, making it a holy portion of the day for self-care and renewal.

Choosing the Right Chair

When practicing chair yoga, especially for men over 50, choosing the proper chair is critical to ensuring the safety and efficacy of the yoga sessions. A decent yoga chair should have a strong, secure base that allows for a variety of exercises without tipping over or sliding. This stability is vital since many positions demand moving body weight in different directions. The chair should not have wheels unless they can be properly fastened to avoid accidental movement during practice.

The height of the chair is another crucial consideration. The perfect chair allows you to sit with your feet firmly planted on the ground and your knees bent at a proper angle. This position aids in the maintenance of good alignment and balance, both of which are required for successfully and safely performing yoga poses. A chair that is too high can strain the lower back and hamstrings, whereas one that is too low can put undue strain on the knees and joints.

The chair's seat should be broad enough to comfortably fit the hips and thighs without compressing them. This provides enough space for mobility and allows you to maintain appropriate posture during your yoga session. However, it should not be so broad that it makes it impossible to reach the floor or maintain proper alignment. The balance between comfort and usefulness is critical.

A chair without arms is often preferable for chair yoga since it provides a wider range of motion. Armrests may hinder the ability to achieve certain postures or transitions effortlessly. Armrests, for example, might make postures that require twisting or extending the arms to the side more difficult. Individuals who require more support, on the other hand, can utilize an arm chair with caution, choosing postures that do not interfere with these structures.

The material of the chair also influences the whole experience. A chair with a small cushion can give comfort when sat, but it should not be too soft to risk stability. Non-slip materials are useful, particularly for the seat, to avoid slipping while changing between positions. Meanwhile, the chair's back should provide support without being too restricting, allowing for flexibility of movement in the upper body.

Durability is another important consideration, since the chair must resist continuous usage over time. Investing in a high-quality chair guarantees that it can withstand the weight and movement involved with yoga sessions without soon wearing out. This not only assures safety, but also that the chair stays a dependable piece of yoga equipment throughout one's practice.

Finally, viewing the chair as an essential component of the yoga practice rather than a mere prop might improve the whole experience. The appropriate chair may make yoga more accessible and pleasurable, allowing those over 50 to participate in a physical practice that promotes strength, flexibility, and mental health. Individuals may safely and efficiently practice chair yoga by carefully selecting a chair that matches these characteristics, making it an important tool for preserving health and energy.

Safety Tips and Modifications

Chair yoga has several benefits for men over 50, including improved flexibility, strength, and mental well-being. However, to guarantee that the practice is both useful and safe, various safeguards and adaptations are required. This is especially crucial as the body ages, making it more prone to injury and longer to heal. Recognizing and accepting your body's present limitations is the first step toward safe practice. It is critical to heed to your body's cues and avoid movements that cause pain or discomfort. Pushing one's limitations can do more harm than good, transforming what should be a caring practice into a source of injury.

When starting chair yoga, choosing the correct chair is critical to ensuring a safe practice. The ideal chair is robust, without wheels, and with a seat that is not overly soft. A chair with a straight back helps to support the spine when seated, and armrests can help with balance and moving in and out of the chair. When seated, make sure your feet can rest flat on the floor; if required, use a block or books to elevate the floor. This improves posture and relieves tension on the legs and lower back.

Warm-ups are an important part of chair yoga, since they prepare the body for more intensive motions. Begin with simple neck rolls, shoulder shrugs, and wrist rotations to lubricate joints and improve blood flow to muscles. These beginning motions should be done slowly and mindfully, to establish a tone of alertness to the body's reactions that will be maintained throughout the session. This awareness aids in determining when a stance is useful and when it is potentially taxing.

Modifications to chair yoga postures guarantee that everyone may practice safely, regardless of flexibility or strength. For example, if a conventional yoga position calls for hands on the floor, utilizing the chair's seat or armrest as a point of contact can provide the same stretch while lowering the danger of overextension. Similarly, straps may be utilized to support postures that require longer reach than is currently accessible, such as leg stretches, without sacrificing form or causing injury.

Breathing is crucial to the safety and efficacy of chair yoga. Deep, regulated breaths serve to oxygenate the body, lower blood pressure, and improve relaxation, resulting in a state of awareness in which one is more aware of the body's powers and limitations. This attention allows for a more introspective practice, with the emphasis on the internal feeling of each position rather than reaching a certain exterior form. Breathing methods are also useful for controlling discomfort or effort, fostering a practice that is guided by one's own breath rather than external expectations.

Balance poses in chair yoga, which are vital for increasing stability and preventing falls, should be approached with caution. Using the chair as support, one may perform standing postures that strengthen the legs and core, which are essential for balance. However, it is critical to do this near a wall or similar solid object to grip onto if balance is lost. Over time, as balance and confidence increase, dependence on these supports can be reduced, with safety always taking precedence over development.

Finally, concluding each chair yoga session with a moment of rest and introspection helps to absorb the practice's benefits and honors the body's efforts. This time can also be utilized to gently evaluate any regions of the body that responded well to the practice or that caused discomfort, which will help guide future sessions. This introspective practice emphasizes the need of progressive growth and personal adaptation in making chair yoga a safe, pleasurable, and helpful activity for men over 50. Through these attentive practices and changes, chair yoga may be a powerful tool for maintaining and developing general health and well-being, adapted to each individual's body's particular demands.

Warm-Up and Cool-Down: Why They Matter

Warm-ups and cool-downs are essential in any physical exercise, particularly chair yoga for men over 50, where safety and efficacy are important. Starting a yoga practice with a warm-up is essential because it prepares the body for the stretches and postures that follow. Warm-up activities, in particular, for men over the age of 50, gently stimulate the muscles, joints, and cardiovascular system, gradually boosting heart rate and blood circulation. This procedure reduces the chance of injury by lubricating the joints and making the muscles more flexible. Warm-ups are necessary to offset these changes and improve mobility because as the body ages, muscles and joints stiffen and become less flexible.

Transitioning into yoga postures from a state of rest without a sufficient warm-up can cause strain and discomfort, especially for individuals who are already suffering with the aches and pains associated with aging. A well-structured warm-up in chair yoga, with an emphasis on gentle stretching and breathing techniques, establishes a good tone for the whole practice. It allows for a more in-depth and thoughtful engagement with yoga postures, resulting in improved comfort and fluidity of movement. This conscious start aids in listening into the body's demands and limitations, promoting a practice that promotes health and well-being rather than pushing the body beyond its comfort zone.

However, it is equally necessary to cool down after a yoga practice. Just as the body must be prepared for the next action, it must also be given the opportunity to appropriately wind down. Cool-down activities in chair yoga, which frequently include slower, deeper stretches and relaxation methods, help the body return to a state of rest. For men over 50, this gradual shift is critical to avoiding rapid fluctuations in blood pressure and heart rate, which may be unsettling and potentially hazardous.

Furthermore, the cool-down period allows you to fully benefit from your yoga practice. It allows the body to absorb the work done throughout the session, which helps to cement the flexibility and strength gains. Relaxation and meditation practices commonly used during the cool-down period provide significant mental health advantages. They promote a condition of awareness and relaxation, which reduces stress and improves general wellbeing.

Focused breathing throughout the warm-up and cool-down periods increases their advantages. Breathwork, or pranayama, is an essential component of yoga that regulates the body's response to physical stress. Mastering breath control can help elderly men enhance respiratory function, boost oxygen flow to their muscles, and promote inner tranquility and focus. This comprehensive approach guarantees that chair yoga is about more than just physical wellness; it is also about cultivating the mind and soul.

The personalized approach of chair yoga, with its emphasis on moderate warm-ups and cool-downs, recognizes the special requirements of men over 50. It acknowledges that the body at this stage of life requires more careful care and a deliberate attitude to physical exercise. By focusing on these qualities, chair yoga becomes an effective tool for preserving and improving physical mobility, strength, and mental clarity far into old age.

Finally, the inclusion of deliberate warm-ups and cool-downs in chair yoga for men over 50 honors the body's wisdom. It's about developing a practice that is both loving and empowering, allowing older men to interact with yoga in ways that benefit their health and happiness. This delicate balance between action and rest, effort and relaxation, is the actual spirit of yoga, making it accessible and useful for persons of any age.

Fundamental Chair Yoga Poses

Seated Mountain Pose

Seated Mountain Pose, or Tadasana in a chair, stands as a foundational pose in chair yoga, especially beneficial for men over 50. This pose is deceptively simple yet profoundly impactful, serving as a cornerstone for establishing good posture, alignment, and awareness of the body's natural state of balance. While it might seem like merely sitting upright, Seated Mountain Pose is an active engagement of muscles, a practice of mindful breathing, and an alignment of body and mind.

Instructions:

- [ ] Begin by sitting at the edge of a sturdy chair, feet planted firmly on the ground, hip-distance apart.
- [ ] Ensure that your knees are directly over your ankles, creating a 90-degree angle with your legs.
- [ ] Root your sit bones evenly into the seat of the chair, engaging your thighs lightly but without tensing up.
- [ ] Straighten your spine, lifting through the crown of your head towards the ceiling, as if a string is gently pulling you upwards.
- [ ] Draw your shoulders back and down, away from your ears, allowing your chest to open and your heart center to lift slightly.
- [ ] Place your hands on your thighs or knees, palms down or up, depending on what feels most comfortable and supportive.
- [ ] Engage your abdominal muscles slightly to support your spine, but maintain natural breathing.
- [ ] Gaze straight ahead, with your chin parallel to the floor, cultivating a sense of dignity and ease within the pose.
- [ ] Hold this pose while taking several deep, steady breaths, focusing on maintaining balance and alignment throughout the body.

☐ To release, simply relax the engagement of your muscles and breathe normally, acknowledging the sense of space and alignment created by the pose.

Benefits:

- **Improves Posture**: Regular practice strengthens the muscles of the back and shoulders, which are crucial for maintaining good posture. This is particularly important for men over 50, as posture tends to decline with age.
- **Enhances Spinal Alignment**: By encouraging the natural curves of the spine, it can alleviate common issues such as back pain and discomfort.
- **Builds Core Strength**: The engagement of the abdominal muscles supports the lower back, promoting core stability and strength.
- **Boosts Circulation**: The upright position helps in improving blood flow, especially beneficial for those spending long hours seated.
- **Reduces Stress**: Focused breathing in this pose promotes relaxation and can help reduce stress and anxiety levels.
- **Increases Awareness**: Practicing this pose fosters a heightened sense of bodily awareness, encouraging mindfulness and a connection between body and mind.
- **Cultivates Balance**: Although seated, the pose teaches balance and grounding, principles that can be applied to other aspects of life and physical activity.

Seated Mountain Pose is a testament to the principle that powerful benefits can come from simple practices. For men over 50, incorporating this pose into their daily routine can be a stepping stone towards improved health, greater awareness, and a balanced approach to life's challenges.

Chair Cat-Cow Stretch

The Chair Cat-Cow Stretch is a foundational pose in chair yoga, especially designed to suit the needs and limitations of men over 50. This gentle yet effective movement sequence offers numerous benefits, making it an essential part of any chair yoga practice for enhancing flexibility, improving posture, and reducing stress.

Instructions:

- ☐ Begin by sitting comfortably towards the front of a sturdy chair, ensuring your feet are flat on the floor and your spine is in a neutral position. Place your hands on your knees or thighs, depending on what feels most comfortable and allows for a full range of motion.

- ☐ Inhale deeply, and as you do, gently arch your back, tilting your pelvis forward. Lift your chest and chin slightly upwards, rolling your shoulders back and away from your ears. This position mirrors the "cow" posture in traditional yoga, adapted for the chair.

- [ ] Hold the cow pose for a few seconds, allowing the stretch to penetrate your chest and throat, while being mindful not to strain your neck.
- [ ] As you exhale, slowly round your spine, tucking your chin to your chest and drawing your belly button towards your spine. Gently lean back just enough to feel a stretch, but not so much that you lose balance. This is the "cat" aspect of the sequence.
- [ ] Maintain the cat pose for a few seconds, feeling the stretch along your spine and across your shoulder blades.
- [ ] Continue to alternate between the Cat and Cow poses for several breath cycles, moving smoothly and slowly. Let your breath guide your movement, with each inhale transitioning into Cow and each exhale into Cat.
- [ ] Focus on the sensation of your spine flexing and extending. This awareness helps in maximizing the stretch and the benefits of the movement.

Benefits:

The Chair Cat-Cow Stretch offers a myriad of benefits, particularly for men over 50, who might be experiencing stiffness, back pain, or reduced mobility.

- **Enhances Spinal Flexibility**: Regular practice of this stretch promotes spinal health, encouraging flexibility and range of motion. It helps combat the stiffness and rigidity that can come with age, making daily activities more comfortable and pain-free.

- **Improves Posture:** By strengthening and stretching the back muscles, this sequence assists in correcting poor posture, a common issue for those who spend a lot of time sitting. A better posture reduces the risk of back and neck pain and improves overall body alignment.

- **Stimulates the Digestive System**: The alternating movement of extending and flexing the torso can help stimulate the abdominal organs, potentially improving digestion and alleviating digestive discomfort.

- **Reduces Stress:** The rhythmic pattern of movement and breathing can have a calming effect on the mind, reducing stress and anxiety levels. The focus required to perform the stretch also aids in mindfulness, bringing a sense of mental clarity and peace.

- **Increases Lung Capacity**: The deep inhalations and exhalations involved in the Cat-Cow Stretch enhance lung capacity and improve respiratory efficiency. This is particularly beneficial for men over 50, as respiratory function can decline with age.

Seated Forward Bend

The Seated Forward Bend, known in traditional yoga as Paschimottanasana, adapts gracefully to chair yoga, making it an accessible and beneficial pose for men over 50. This variation takes into account the common physical limitations and safety concerns of older adults, while still offering the core benefits of the pose. In chair yoga, the Seated Forward Bend focuses on stretching the spine, shoulders, and hamstrings, promoting flexibility and relieving tension in these areas.

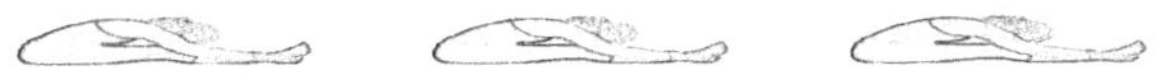

Instructions:

☐ Begin by sitting at the edge of a sturdy chair, feet planted firmly on the ground, hip-distance apart.

- [ ] Keep your spine long and your hands resting on your thighs. Inhale deeply.
- [ ] As you exhale, hinge at your hips and slowly bend forward, allowing your hands to slide down your legs toward your feet.
- [ ] Go only as far as comfortable, keeping your back straight rather than rounded. Your goal is to feel a stretch in your back and hamstrings, not to reach your toes.
- [ ] Let your head hang gently, releasing tension in your neck and shoulders.
- [ ] Hold the position for several breaths, deepening the stretch with each exhale.
- [ ] To come out of the pose, inhale and gently raise your torso, using your hands on your thighs for support, returning to a seated position.

Benefits:

The Seated Forward Bend offers numerous physical and mental benefits, particularly valuable for men over 50. Physically, it stretches the spine, shoulders, and hamstrings. This stretching can alleviate stiffness and pain, which are common issues as the body ages. Improved flexibility in these areas can lead to better posture and mobility, reducing the risk of falls and injuries.

This pose also stimulates the abdominal organs, which can aid digestion and alleviate problems like constipation. For men dealing with the stresses of daily life, the forward bend encourages a moment of introspection and mental relaxation, providing a break from external stimuli and allowing for a moment of calm. The action of bending forward can also help reduce anxiety and fatigue by promoting a sense of letting go and surrendering burdens, both physical and mental.

By enhancing circulation, the Seated Forward Bend ensures better blood flow throughout the body. This is particularly beneficial for heart health, as increased circulation supports the cardiovascular system. Moreover, the pose encourages deeper breathing, which improves oxygenation to the body's tissues, supports respiratory function, and enhances overall energy levels.

Chair Extended Side Angle

The Chair Extended Side Angle Pose is a modified version of the traditional Extended Side Angle Pose, adapted for chair yoga to make it accessible and beneficial for men over 50. This adaptation allows individuals to experience the pose's benefits without the need for extensive flexibility or balance, making it ideal for those who are new to yoga, recovering from injury, or dealing with chronic conditions that affect their mobility.

Instructions:

- [ ] Begin by sitting sideways on a sturdy chair, ensuring that your right side is facing the back of the chair. Keep your feet flat on the floor, hip-width apart.
- [ ] Turn your right foot out so that it points directly towards the back of the chair, and keep your left foot

firmly planted on the ground, toes pointing forward. Align your knees with your feet.

- [ ] Place your right hand on the back of the chair. This will be your support as you move into the pose.
- [ ] Inhale deeply, and as you exhale, gently hinge at your hips, leaning your torso to the right, and extend your left arm up and over your head, creating a straight line from your left foot up through your left fingertips. Your right arm can remain on the chair for support, or if you feel stable, you can lower it towards the floor to deepen the stretch.
- [ ] Keep your chest open and facing forward, rather than down towards the floor. This helps to increase the stretch across your chest and shoulders.
- [ ] Hold the pose for several deep breaths, aiming for a gentle stretch along your left side. With each exhale, try to deepen the stretch slightly, but be mindful not to push too hard.
- [ ] To come out of the pose, use your right hand to push yourself back up to a seated position. Repeat on the other side by turning to face the opposite side of the chair and following the same steps.

Benefits:

The Chair Extended Side Angle Pose offers a myriad of benefits, especially tailored to the needs of men over 50. Some of the key benefits include:

- **Improved Flexibility**: This pose stretches the side of the body, from the ankles to the fingertips, improving flexibility in the spine, waist, and shoulders.
- **Enhanced Respiratory Function**: By opening the chest and sides of the body, this pose encourages deeper breathing, which can enhance lung capacity and improve respiratory function.
- **Strengthening**: It strengthens the legs, particularly the thighs, by maintaining a seated position that requires muscle engagement.
- **Reduced Back Pain**: By stretching the spine and opening the hips, this pose can help alleviate back pain, a common issue for men over 50.
- **Increased Circulation**: The side stretch encourages blood flow throughout the body, which can improve overall circulation and contribute to cardiovascular health.
- **Stress Relief**: The focused breathing and gentle stretching help to relieve stress and promote a sense of calm and well-being.
- **Better Balance and Stability**: Although the pose is performed seated, it requires and thus develops a sense of

balance and stability, which are crucial for preventing falls.

The Chair Extended Side Angle Pose demonstrates how chair yoga can be adapted to meet the needs of older adults, providing them with a safe and effective way to enjoy the benefits of yoga. This pose, in particular, offers a balanced approach to physical fitness, combining strength, flexibility, and mental relaxation, making it a valuable addition to any yoga practice for men over 50.

Seated Spinal Twist

The Seated Spinal Twist is a cornerstone pose in chair yoga, particularly beneficial for men over 50. This pose, known for its simplicity and adaptability, offers a multitude of health benefits, especially for those seeking to maintain or enhance their physical and mental well-being as they age. It involves twisting the torso while seated, which can help to increase spinal mobility, improve digestion, and reduce back pain—a common complaint among older adults.

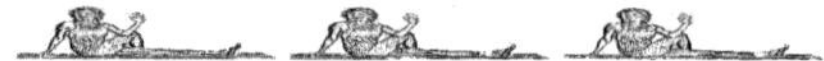

Instructions:

- [ ] Begin by sitting sideways on a chair, ensuring that your feet are flat on the floor and your spine is elongated. If your feet don't comfortably reach the ground, consider using a block or a small stool to support your feet.
- [ ] Place your hands on the back of the chair. For a right-side twist, your left hand should be on the chair's right side, and your right hand should be on the chair's back.

- [ ] Inhale deeply, and as you exhale, gently twist your torso to the right, using your hands for support to deepen the twist. Keep your spine tall and your chin aligned with your shoulder.
- [ ] Hold the position for a few breaths, focusing on deepening the twist slightly with each exhale without straining. It's important to listen to your body and not push beyond a comfortable stretch.
- [ ] To return to the starting position, use an inhale to slowly untwist your torso, facing forward once again.
- [ ] Repeat the twist on the opposite side to ensure balance in the stretch. If you began by twisting to the right, rotate your chair to perform the twist to the left.
- [ ] Throughout the pose, keep your shoulders relaxed and away from your ears, and ensure your movements are slow and controlled to avoid any sudden strain on the back or spine.

Benefits:

1. **Improved Spinal Flexibility**: Regularly practicing this twist can enhance the flexibility of the spine. As men age, the spine can become stiff and less mobile, leading to discomfort and reduced range of motion. This pose helps combat that stiffness, promoting better posture and movement.

2. **Enhanced Digestive Health**: The twisting motion massages the abdominal organs, stimulating digestion and helping to alleviate issues like bloating and constipation. This gentle pressure and release can improve overall gastrointestinal function.

3. **Stress Reduction**: Twisting poses are known for their ability to release tension in the spine and back, areas where many people hold stress. By engaging in this gentle twist, men can experience a reduction in stress and anxiety levels, contributing to better mental health.

4. **Increased Circulation**: The act of twisting and then releasing helps to encourage blood flow throughout the torso, nourishing the spinal discs and muscles. Improved circulation can lead to faster recovery from injuries and can help in reducing inflammation.

5. **Detoxification**: The compression and release inherent in twisting poses are thought to help with the body's natural detoxification processes, aiding in the removal of toxins and encouraging the flow of fresh nutrients to the tissues.

6. **Balance and Coordination**: As a balance-focused pose, the Seated Spinal Twist aids in improving one's sense of body awareness and coordination, which are crucial for preventing falls and maintaining independence.

The Seated Spinal Twist is a versatile pose that can be easily adapted to accommodate different levels of mobility and flexibility, making it an ideal practice for men over 50. Its benefits extend beyond physical well-being, offering men a tool for managing stress and enhancing their overall quality of life. As with any yoga practice, it's important to proceed gently and consult with a healthcare provider if there are any concerns about injuries or physical conditions.

Seated Warrior Poses

Seated Warrior Poses in chair yoga offer a fantastic way for men over 50 to engage in yoga practice safely and effectively. These poses, adapted to be performed while seated, provide many of the same benefits as their standing counterparts but are more accessible for those with balance issues, joint concerns, or limited mobility. They are designed to strengthen the body, enhance flexibility, and promote mental focus.

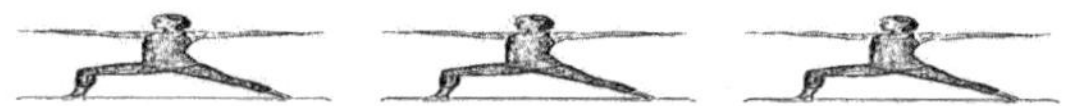

Seated Warrior I Pose

- [ ] Begin by sitting on the edge of a sturdy chair, feet flat on the floor, and legs hip-width apart.

- [ ] Extend your right leg back, keeping your right foot on the ground and your leg straight. Your body will be facing forward, with this pose focusing on stretching the hip flexors and engaging the core.
- [ ] Inhale and raise your arms above your head, keeping them parallel to each other with palms facing inward.
- [ ] Gently arch your back and look up, engaging your core to maintain balance. Hold this position for several breaths, focusing on the stretch and strength being built.
- [ ] Exhale and slowly lower your arms, returning to the starting position. Repeat on the other side.

Seated Warrior II Pose

- [ ] From the same starting position as Warrior I, extend your right leg to the side, keeping your left foot directly under your left knee.
- [ ] Turn your torso to the right, extending your arms out to the sides at shoulder height, palms facing down. Your head turns to look over your right hand, aligning the pose and focusing on the extension through both arms.
- [ ] This pose emphasizes the engagement of the thigh muscles while keeping the hips facing forward. Hold for several breaths, feeling the stretch along your arms and the engagement in your legs.

☐ To release, gently lower your arms and return to the starting position before repeating on the opposite side.

Benefits of Seated Warrior Poses

1. **Strengthens Muscles:** These poses target the core, thighs, and arms, helping to build strength in these essential areas. This is particularly beneficial for men over 50, as maintaining muscle mass is crucial for overall health and mobility.

2. Improves Flexibility and Mobility: Regular practice of seated warrior poses can enhance flexibility in the hips and shoulders, areas often tight in men over 50. Increased mobility helps in daily activities and can reduce the risk of falls.

3. Enhances Mental Focus: Holding the poses requires concentration and breath control, which can improve mental focus and reduce stress. The practice encourages mindfulness, connecting the body's movements with the breath.

4. Promotes Better Posture: These poses engage the core and back muscles, which are vital for good posture. Improved posture can alleviate common issues like back pain and neck stiffness.

5. Encourages Joint Health: By moving the joints through their range of motion, these poses support joint flexibility and can help reduce stiffness and pain, common concerns for men over 50.

Incorporating seated warrior poses into a chair yoga routine offers a balanced approach to physical and mental well-being for men over 50. These poses are a testament to the adaptability of yoga, proving that with modifications, the practice is accessible and beneficial for individuals at any stage of life, promoting strength, flexibility, and peace of mind.

Strength Building with Chair Yoga

Seated Chair Sun Salutations

Seated Chair Sun Salutations offer a modified version of the traditional Sun Salutations, specifically tailored to build strength, improve flexibility, and enhance the overall well-being of men over 50 through chair yoga. This adaptation allows individuals to experience the flow and benefits of Sun Salutations while seated, making it accessible for those with mobility concerns, balance issues, or anyone who finds standing exercises challenging.

The sequence combines gentle yet effective movements coordinated with breath, designed to warm up the body, stimulate the cardiovascular system, and strengthen major muscle groups.

Here's a step-by-step guide to performing Seated Chair Sun Salutations:

1. Start in Seated Mountain Pose: Sit at the edge of a sturdy chair with your feet flat on the floor, hip-width apart. Engage your core, straighten your spine, and place your hands on your knees. Take a deep breath in and out, establishing your starting position.

2. Upward Salute: Inhale and sweep your arms out to the sides and up overhead. Bring your palms together, if possible, gazing up toward your hands, keeping your shoulders down away from your ears. This movement helps to stretch the sides of the body and mobilizes the shoulders.

3. Forward Bend: Exhale, and hinge at your hips to fold forward, lowering your hands towards your feet. Allow your torso to come down as close to your legs as comfortable, promoting flexibility in the spine and hamstrings.

4. Halfway Lift: Inhale, and lift your torso up halfway, lengthening your spine forward. Place your hands on your knees or shins. This pose strengthens the back muscles and encourages a neutral spine.

5. Forward Fold then Seated Upward Salute: Exhale and fold forward again. Then, inhale, sweeping your arms wide to the sides and overhead, returning to the Upward Salute.

6. Chair Pose: Exhale, and bring your arms down, bending your elbows to a 90-degree angle as if sitting back into an imaginary chair further behind you. This strengthens the shoulders, arms, and core, and engages the thighs as if you're about to stand, offering a gentle cardiovascular boost.

7. Return to Seated Mountain Pose: Inhale, straightening your arms up overhead again. Exhale, bringing your

hands to prayer position at your heart, then release your hands to your knees, returning to Seated Mountain Pose.

8. Repeat this sequence several times, ideally 3-5 rounds, to fully experience its benefits.

Benefits:

- **Improved Flexibility**: Regularly performing this sequence can enhance flexibility, particularly in the spine, shoulders, and hamstrings, areas where men over 50 often experience stiffness.

- **Increased Strength:** This sequence engages major muscle groups, including the core, arms, and legs, building strength in a balanced way that supports daily activities.

- **Enhanced Cardiovascular Health**: The rhythmic nature of Sun Salutations, even when seated, can help increase heart rate slightly, promoting cardiovascular health.

- **Stress Reduction**: The coordination of movement and breath helps focus the mind, reducing stress and promoting mental clarity.

- **Better Posture**: The emphasis on spine alignment and core engagement helps improve posture, which can alleviate common aches and pains associated with poor posture.

- **Increased Joint Health**: Gentle movements increase circulation to the joints, helping to reduce discomfort and promote mobility.

By integrating Seated Chair Sun Salutations into their routine, men over 50 can enjoy a comprehensive exercise that not only builds physical strength but also enhances mental well-being, making it a cornerstone of a holistic approach to health in later life.

Chair Plank Variations

Chair yoga offers a unique and accessible way for men over 50 to build strength, focusing on safe practices that cater to their needs. Among the various exercises, chair plank variations stand out for their adaptability and effectiveness in enhancing core strength, stability, and overall muscular endurance. These variations provide a low-impact alternative to traditional planks, reducing strain on the wrists and shoulders, which is particularly beneficial for those who may have joint issues or are new to strength training.

Seated Chair Plank Variation:

- [ ] Begin by sitting at the edge of a sturdy chair, feet flat on the ground, and knees bent at a 90-degree angle.
- [ ] Place your hands on either side of the chair seat, ensuring they are directly under your shoulders.
- [ ] Engage your core and lift your hips off the chair, moving your feet slightly forward so your body forms a straight line from your head to your knees.
- [ ] Hold this position, keeping your core engaged and breathing deeply. Aim to maintain the pose for 15 to 30 seconds, then slowly lower your hips back to the starting position.

Chair Plank with Leg Lift Variation:

- [ ] Start in the seated chair plank position.
- [ ] Once stable, slowly lift one foot off the ground, extending the leg straight out in front of you, while keeping your core engaged.
- [ ] Hold the lift for a few seconds, then gently place the foot back on the ground.
- [ ] Repeat with the other leg. Aim for 5 to 10 lifts per leg, focusing on maintaining form and balance.

Standing Chair Plank Variation:

- [ ] Stand facing the chair, placing your hands on the top of the backrest. Step back until your body forms a diagonal line from your heels to your head.
- [ ] Engage your core, ensuring your body remains straight and strong. Your arms should be straight, with shoulders directly above your wrists.
- [ ] Hold this position, focusing on keeping your body as rigid and straight as a plank. Aim for 15 to 30 seconds, then carefully walk your feet towards the chair to release the pose.

Benefits of Chair Plank Variations:

1. **Improved Core Strength**: These exercises engage the entire core, including the abdominals, obliques, and lower back muscles, leading to improved core stability and strength.

2. **Enhanced Upper Body Strength**: By using the chair for support, these plank variations also work the shoulders, chest, and arms, helping to build upper body strength without heavy lifting.

3. **Increased Balance and Stability**: Regular practice of chair plank variations can improve balance and stability, which are crucial for preventing falls and maintaining independence.

4. **Joint-Friendly**: For men over 50, especially those with joint concerns or arthritis, chair plank variations offer a lower-impact option for strength training, reducing the risk of injury.

5. **Versatility and Accessibility**: These variations can be easily adjusted to fit individual fitness levels, making them suitable for beginners and those with limited mobility.

6. **Mental Focus**: Holding a plank requires concentration and breath control, which can help improve mental focus and reduce stress.

Incorporating chair plank variations into a regular chair yoga practice provides a safe and effective way for men over 50 to enhance their physical strength and overall well-being. These exercises demonstrate that with the right adaptations, anyone can enjoy the benefits of strength training, regardless of age or fitness level.

Seated Leg Lifts and Extensions

Seated leg lifts and extensions are a cornerstone exercise in chair yoga, particularly beneficial for men over 50 looking to build strength, enhance flexibility, and improve balance without the risk of strain or injury associated with standing workouts. This exercise, tailored for a seated position, targets the muscles of the lower body, including the quadriceps, hamstrings, and core, offering a safe and effective way to maintain muscle tone and support joint health.

Instructions:

- [ ] Begin by sitting upright in a sturdy chair that doesn't have arms, ensuring your feet are flat on the ground. Place your hands on the sides of the chair for stability. This starting position helps promote good posture and alignment, which are crucial for the effective execution of the exercise.

- [ ] Engage your core muscles to provide support for your lower back. This engagement is key to stabilizing your torso and preventing any undue strain as you move through the exercise.

- [ ] Slowly lift one leg at a time, keeping the knee straight but not locked. Elevate the leg to a height that feels challenging yet manageable, aiming for parallel to the floor if possible. The act of lifting the leg engages the quadriceps, the major muscle group at the front of the thigh.

- ☐ Hold the lifted position for a count of three to five seconds. This isometric hold increases muscle endurance and strength by challenging the muscles to maintain the position under tension.

- ☐ Gently lower the leg back to the starting position, controlling the movement to maximize the engagement of the muscles throughout the entire range of motion.

- ☐ After completing the desired number of repetitions with one leg, switch to the other leg and repeat the process. This ensures balanced strength development across both sides of the body.

- ☐ For an added challenge and to target the hamstrings and glutes, consider extending the leg straight out and then flexing the foot to bring the heel towards you in a controlled manner before lowering the leg. This variation not only strengthens but also enhances flexibility in the leg muscles.

Benefits:

Seated leg lifts and extensions offer numerous benefits for men over 50 engaging in chair yoga. Firstly, they strengthen the quadriceps, hamstrings, and calves, which are vital for everyday activities such as walking, climbing stairs, and rising from a seated position. Stronger leg muscles contribute to better support of the knee and hip joints, potentially reducing the risk of pain and injury.

Moreover, this exercise engages the core muscles, including the abdominals and the lower back. A strong core is essential for maintaining good posture, reducing lower back pain, and improving balance, which can decrease the likelihood of falls—a common concern among older adults.

The controlled movement and breathing associated with seated leg lifts and extensions also enhance proprioception, or the body's ability to sense its position in space. Improved proprioception supports better coordination and agility, contributing to a higher quality of life.

Additionally, incorporating these exercises into a regular chair yoga routine can lead to improvements in flexibility and range of motion. The act of lifting and extending the legs stretches the muscles, making daily movements more fluid and less restrictive.

Finally, seated leg lifts and extensions can have a positive impact on mental health. The focus required to perform the exercise mindfully helps cultivate concentration and reduces stress, promoting a sense of well-being that extends beyond the physical benefits of the exercise.

Seated leg lifts and extensions are an invaluable component of chair yoga for men over 50, offering a holistic approach to strength building that supports both physical and mental health. By integrating these exercises into their routine, individuals can enjoy improved muscle tone, joint health, balance, and overall well-being.

Improving Flexibility

Gentle Seated Stretches

Gentle seated stretches in chair yoga offer a safe and effective way for men over 50 to improve flexibility, reduce stiffness, and enhance overall well-being. These stretches are designed to be accessible, focusing on slowly lengthening the muscles and increasing the range of motion in a controlled manner. By incorporating these stretches into their routine, individuals can experience significant health benefits, including improved posture, decreased back pain, and a reduction in the risk of injury. Here's a look at some key gentle seated stretches, along with instructions and their benefits.

1. **Seated Forward Bend:** This stretch targets the spine, shoulders, and hamstrings. Begin by sitting at the edge of your chair with feet flat on the ground. Inhale deeply, and as you exhale, slowly hinge at the hips, lowering your torso towards your thighs. Extend your hands towards your feet, keeping the spine long. Hold this position for a few breaths, then gently return to the starting position. This stretch aids in relieving tension in the back and legs and improves flexibility in the hamstrings and lower back.

2. **Seated Cat-Cow Stretch**: Ideal for improving spinal flexibility and relieving tension in the back. Sit with your feet flat and hands on your knees. Inhale, arch your back, and look up towards the ceiling for the cow position. Exhale, round your spine, tucking your chin to your chest for the cat position. Alternate between these two positions, moving with your breath. This stretch enhances spinal mobility and can help alleviate back pain.

3. **Seated Spinal Twist**: This stretch targets the spine, shoulders, and neck. Sit up straight with your feet flat on the floor. Place your right hand on the back of the chair and your left hand on your right knee. As you inhale, lengthen your spine, and as you exhale, gently twist to the right, looking over your right shoulder. Hold for a few breaths, then return to center and repeat on the other side. The spinal twist improves spinal flexibility and can aid in digestion.

4. **Chair Pigeon Pose**: Focuses on the hips, glutes, and lower back. While seated, place your right ankle on your left knee, forming a figure 4. Keep your back straight, and gently lean forward to deepen the stretch. Hold for several breaths, then switch sides. This pose is excellent for opening up the hips and relieving tightness in the lower back.

5. **Neck and Shoulder Stretch**: Helps to relieve tension in the neck, shoulders, and upper back. Sit upright and gently tilt your head to the right, bringing your ear

towards your shoulder. For a deeper stretch, place your right hand on your head and apply gentle pressure. Hold for a few breaths, then repeat on the other side. For the shoulders, roll them slowly forwards and backwards, then stretch one arm across your body, using the other arm to press it towards your chest.

They are especially beneficial for men over 50, as flexibility tends to decrease with age, leading to stiffness, reduced mobility, and a higher risk of injuries. Regularly practicing these stretches can improve range of motion, reduce pain and stiffness, and enhance the quality of life by making daily activities easier and more comfortable. Additionally, the mindful nature of chair yoga and its focus on breathwork can also contribute to reduced stress and improved mental clarity, making it a holistic practice beneficial for both body and mind.

Shoulder and Neck Release

Shoulder and neck tension is a common issue among men over 50, often resulting from prolonged periods of sitting, poor posture, or the natural process of aging. Chair yoga offers an effective way to address these concerns, promoting flexibility and relief through gentle, accessible exercises. By focusing on shoulder and neck release, chair yoga can alleviate discomfort, enhance mobility, and contribute to overall well-being. The practices detailed below are designed with the older practitioner in mind, providing a safe and supportive approach to improving flexibility in these critical areas.

- **Seated Mountain Pose with Shoulder Rolls**: Begin in a seated mountain pose, sitting upright in your chair with feet flat on the floor. Inhale deeply and, as you exhale, roll your shoulders slowly forward, up towards your ears, and then back, creating a circular motion. Repeat this movement 5-10 times, then reverse the direction. This exercise helps to loosen the shoulder joints and reduce tension in the surrounding muscles.

- **Neck Side Stretch**: Remain seated with your spine long and your feet planted on the ground. Place your right hand over your head so that your palm rests gently on the left ear. Gently pull your head towards your right shoulder, keeping your left shoulder down. Hold for 15-30 seconds, feeling a stretch on the left side of your neck. Repeat on the other side. This stretch alleviates tightness in the neck muscles and enhances lateral flexibility.

- **Chin Tuck**: Sit up straight and look forward. Without nodding or tilting your head, pull your chin straight back, creating a "double chin." Hold this position for 3-5 seconds and then release. Repeat 5-10 times. This exercise strengthens the neck muscles and helps in releasing tension in the neck and upper back.

- **Seated Cat-Cow Stretch**: Place your hands on your knees. As you inhale, arch your back and tilt your head slightly back, pushing your chest forward (cow position). As you exhale, round your spine, tucking your chin to your chest and pulling your belly in (cat position). Move smoothly between these two positions for 5-10 cycles. This movement enhances spinal flexibility and releases tension in the shoulders and neck.

- **Eagle Arms**: Stretch your arms straight in front of your body at shoulder height. Cross your right arm over your left, bending at the elbows to bring your palms to touch, or as close as possible. Lift the elbows while dropping the shoulders away from the ears. Hold for 15-30 seconds to stretch the shoulders and upper back, then switch sides. This pose is excellent for releasing deep-seated tension in the shoulders and improving mobility.

- **Shoulder Blade Squeeze**: Sit up tall in your chair, arms by your sides. Inhale and as you exhale, draw your shoulder blades towards each other, as if trying to hold a pencil between them. Hold this squeeze for 3-5 seconds, then release. Repeat 5-10 times. This exercise helps in correcting posture by strengthening the muscles of the upper back and releasing tension in the shoulders.

- **Neck Rotation**: With your spine straight, slowly turn your head to the right, aiming to look over your shoulder without straining. Hold for a few seconds, then gently rotate to the left side. Keep the movement smooth and avoid pushing beyond your comfortable range of motion. This enhances neck flexibility and reduces stiffness.

The benefits of these chair yoga exercises for shoulder and neck release are multifaceted. Regular practice can lead to a significant reduction in pain and stiffness, making daily activities more comfortable and enjoyable. Improved flexibility in the shoulders and neck also contributes to better posture, which can alleviate common issues like headaches and upper back pain. Moreover, these exercises promote relaxation and stress reduction, as releasing physical tension often leads to mental and emotional relief. For men over 50, integrating shoulder and neck release exercises into a chair yoga routine is a practical and effective strategy for maintaining and enhancing quality of life through improved flexibility and well-being.

Hip and Groin Openers

Improving flexibility, particularly around the hip and groin areas, is crucial for men over 50 to maintain mobility, reduce pain, and enhance the quality of life. As we age, our hips and groin can become tight due to prolonged periods of sitting and reduced physical activity, leading to discomfort and limited range of motion. Chair yoga offers a gentle yet effective way to address these concerns, with specific poses designed to open up these areas, increasing flexibility and decreasing discomfort.

Hip and Groin Openers in Chair Yoga

One of the fundamental poses for opening the hips and groin is the Seated Wide Leg Stretch. This pose gently stretches the inner thighs, hips, and groin, promoting flexibility and circulation in these areas.

- [ ] Begin by sitting on the edge of a sturdy chair with your feet planted firmly on the ground.
- [ ] Slowly separate your legs as wide as comfortable, keeping your feet on the ground and your spine straight.
- [ ] Place your hands on your thighs or knees and, with a straight back, hinge forward from your hips, leading with your chest.

☐ Hold this position, breathing deeply for several breaths, then gently come back to the starting position.

Another beneficial pose is the Seated Pigeon Pose, which targets the hip flexors and can help relieve tightness in the lower back.

☐ Sit on the chair with your feet flat on the ground and spine erect.

☐ Carefully lift your right ankle and place it on your left thigh, just above the knee, creating a figure-4 shape with your legs.

☐ Keeping your back straight, gently lean forward to deepen the stretch. You should feel a stretch in your right hip and outer thigh.

☐ Hold for several breaths, then slowly release and switch sides.

The Chair Warrior II Pose is also excellent for opening the hips and strengthening the legs.

☐ Stand behind the chair, using the back of the chair for support if needed.

☐ Step your right foot forward and your left foot back, turning your left foot out about 45 degrees.

☐ Bend your right knee, ensuring it doesn't go past your toes, while keeping your left leg straight.

☐ Extend your arms out to the sides, parallel to the floor, and gaze over your right hand.

☐ Hold this pose for several breaths, feeling the stretch in your hips and groin, then switch sides.

Benefits of Hip and Groin Openers

Practicing these chair yoga poses offers numerous benefits for men over 50, including:

- **Increased Flexibility:** Regularly performing hip and groin openers helps increase the range of motion, making daily activities easier and more comfortable.

- **Reduced Lower Back Pain:** Tight hips often contribute to lower back pain. By opening the hips, there's a decrease in tension and discomfort in the lower back area.

- **Improved Circulation:** These stretches help improve blood flow to the lower body, which can reduce swelling and promote healing in the legs and feet.

- **Enhanced Posture:** Tight hips can lead to poor posture. Hip openers can help align the pelvis, improving posture and reducing strain on the spine.

- **Stress Relief:** Focusing on the breath while engaging in these poses can have a calming effect on the mind, reducing stress and promoting relaxation.

Enhancing Balance and Stability

Chair-Assisted Standing Poses

Chair-assisted standing poses form a core component of chair yoga, particularly beneficial for men over 50 seeking to enhance their balance and stability. As the body ages, maintaining balance becomes increasingly challenging, yet it's essential for daily activities and preventing falls. Chair yoga offers a safe, effective way to improve balance through gentle, supported exercises. Here's a closer look at how chair-assisted standing poses can be integrated into a routine, including detailed instructions and the benefits they offer.

Chair-Assisted Tree Pose

Instructions:

- ☐ Stand with the back of a chair facing you, holding onto the chair's backrest for support.
- ☐ Shift your weight onto your right foot, grounding through the sole while slightly bending your left knee.
- ☐ Place the sole of your left foot on the inner calf or ankle of your standing leg, avoiding the knee joint.

- [ ] Focus on a fixed point in front of you to help maintain balance.
- [ ] Hold the pose for 5-10 breaths, then switch sides.
- [ ] **Benefits**: This pose strengthens the thighs, calves, ankles, and spine while improving overall balance and focus. The support of the chair allows for gradual progression in balance capability.

Chair-Assisted Warrior I

Instructions:

- [ ] Stand with the chair to your side and your hand on the backrest for support.
- [ ] Step your right foot forward and your left foot back, keeping both feet pointed forward or the back foot slightly outward.
- [ ] Bend your front knee, ensuring it does not go past your toes, while keeping your back leg straight.
- [ ] Raise your free arm towards the ceiling or keep it on your hip, depending on your balance.
- [ ] Hold for several breaths, focusing on stretching and stabilizing, then switch sides.
- [ ] **Benefits**: Enhances lower body strength, particularly in the legs and ankles, and increases spinal flexibility. It also improves focus and stamina.

Chair-Assisted Forward Fold

Instructions:

- [ ] Stand facing the chair, feet hip-width apart.
- [ ] Hinge at your hips to fold forward, placing your hands on the chair's seat or backrest, depending on your flexibility.
- [ ] Let your head and neck relax, feeling a stretch along your spine and legs.
- [ ] Hold this position for 5-10 breaths, gently coming back up to stand.
- [ ] Benefits: This pose stretches the spine, shoulders, and hamstrings, providing relief from tension and improving circulation. It also aids in calming the mind and enhancing body awareness.

Chair-Assisted Side Angle Pose

Instructions:

- [ ] Stand with the chair on your right side, holding the backrest for support.
- [ ] Step your right foot out to the side, bending your knee directly over your ankle.

- [ ] Extend your left leg back, keeping your foot flat and angled slightly outward.
- [ ] Lean your torso to the right, placing your right forearm on the chair's seat or backrest.
- [ ] Extend your left arm overhead, stretching through the side of your body.
- [ ] Hold for several breaths, then switch sides.
- [ ] **Benefits**: Improves flexibility in the sides of the body and strengthens the legs. It also aids in opening the hips and improving lung capacity through the side stretch.

Balance-Enhancing Techniques

Balance-enhancing methods are a cornerstone of chair yoga for men over 50, fostering not just physical stability but also a feeling of mental and emotional harmony. This component of yoga practice is especially important for older persons, since keeping balance may improve one's quality of life by lowering the danger of falls and the dread that comes with them. Chair yoga provides a safe and accessible way to enhance balance via a series of modified postures and practices that focus on strengthening the muscles that support stability, improving proprioception, and building a deeper connection between the body and mind.

One of the most basic ways for improving balance in chair yoga is to utilize the chair as a support for stability while practicing standing or seated postures. This strategy allows people to focus on proper muscular alignment and activation without fear of falling. For example, in a chair-assisted tree pose, practitioners can stand with one hand on the back of the chair and the sole of one foot on the inner thigh of the opposite leg, allowing them to securely practice balance on one leg. This activity gradually develops the ankles, calves, thighs, and core muscles, all of which are necessary for balance.

Another strategy focuses on proprioception, which is the body's capacity to detect its own location in space. Chair yoga improves this feeling by requiring the practitioner to shift postures slowly and deliberately, such as raising one foot off the ground while seated or standing behind the chair and taking one step back at a time. These motions urge the practitioner to pay great attention to their body's feelings, which improves their capacity to modify their posture and placement to stay balanced.

Breathwork, or pranayama, is also essential for improving balance in chair yoga. Controlled breathing techniques assist to relax the mind, reduce anxiety, and focus attention, all of which are necessary for maintaining physical equilibrium. Men over 50 can improve their yoga practice by learning to breathe deeply and evenly, especially during demanding positions.

Another important part of chair yoga balancing methods is core strength. The core muscles, which include the belly, lower back, hips, and pelvis, are essential for maintaining overall body stability. Chair yoga contains poses and activities that activate and develop these muscles, such as sitting twists, forward bends, and side stretches, resulting in better balance and posture.

Drishti, or visual concentration, is a yoga method that involves focusing one's eyes on a single place to improve balance. This activity helps to reduce distractions and improve attention, both of which are essential for maintaining balance. Chair yoga practitioners are frequently urged to keep their attention fixed on a stationary object while executing balance poses, which improves stability and mental clarity.

Additionally, practicing transitions between positions in chair yoga improves balance. Moving slowly and thoughtfully from one posture to the next, supported by the chair, helps older persons gain confidence in their ability to maintain balance while moving. This is especially significant in everyday situations when stability during transitions, such as rising up from a seated posture, is required.

In conclusion, chair yoga for men over 50 contains a variety of balance-enhancing methods that are critical for strengthening stability, reducing falls, and instilling confidence in one's physical skills. Chair yoga provides a holistic approach to balance for older individuals by including props, concentrated breathwork, proprioceptive exercises, core strengthening, visual attention, and mindful transitions. This holistic discipline not only improves bodily balance, but also adds to general well-being and a more active, joyful lifestyle.

Integrating Breath and Movement for Better Balance

In chair yoga, which is specifically intended for men over 50, combining breath with movement is a core element that improves balance and stability, both of which are critical components of sustaining a healthy and active lifestyle in later life. This integration, which is strongly established in the practice of yoga, goes beyond simple physical movement by tapping into the body's innate rhythms and the mind's ability to focus and quiet. As men age, the need of balance grows, with stability being critical to performing everyday tasks and avoiding falls.

In yoga, breath, also known as pranayama, is the life energy that energizes and revitalizes the body. Chair yoga synchronizes breathing methods with movements, resulting in a smooth flow that improves coordination and mental alertness. This synchrony helps to stabilize the core muscles, which are essential for maintaining posture and balance. For men over 50, whose stability may be weakened by the natural aging process or sedentary lifestyles, practicing breath-coordinated movements can considerably enhance their feeling of balance.

The process of focusing on the breath while moving through various chair yoga postures promotes a higher level of attention, which enhances balance. Mindfulness fosters a greater understanding of the body's location in space and motions, allowing for rapid and subtle modifications to maintain balance. This is especially useful for older men because it educates the body to adapt more effectively to anticipated balance issues, lowering the chance of falling.

Furthermore, combining breath and movement has a relaxing impact on the neurological system, lowering anxiety and tension, which can impair balance. Stress tightens muscles and can cause a distracted mind, both of which are bad for stability. Focused breathing relaxes the body, loosens the muscles, and clears the mind, all of which lead to improved balance. This relaxing impact can also enhance sleep quality and mood in men over 50, adding to their sense of balance and stability.

Chair yoga positions that include breath work, such as the sitting mountain pose with synchronized arm lifts or the chair warrior pose with concentrated inhalations and exhalations, are especially meant to develop the core and leg muscles. These muscles are essential for balance, and strengthening them via chair yoga practices results in a more firm and confident posture in both yoga and daily life.

Integrating breath and movement increases proprioception, the body's capacity to detect movement, activity, and position. It is a necessary component of equilibrium, especially since sensory capacities may deteriorate with aging. Men over the age of 50 can better navigate their surroundings by improving their proprioception, which allows them to modify their posture and movement to prevent falls and maintain stability.

Finally, the integration of breath and movement in chair yoga provides a comprehensive approach to improving balance and stability in men over 50. This technique not only improves the physical body, but it also relaxes the mind and fosters a stronger bond between them. As balance and stability improve, men over 50 can live a more active, independent, and confident life. Chair yoga, with its emphasis on breath-coordinated movements, becomes not simply a kind of exercise, but a gateway to total well-being and increased life experience in the latter years.

Relaxation and Stress Reduction

Guided Breathing Exercises

Guided breathing exercises are a core component of chair yoga, particularly beneficial for men over 50, aiming to enhance relaxation and reduce stress. These exercises, when performed regularly, can significantly improve physical health, mental clarity, and emotional well-being. For men in this age group, who may be facing increased stress, health issues, or the challenges of aging, incorporating guided breathing exercises into their yoga practice offers a practical and accessible way to foster relaxation and manage stress levels.

One of the most fundamental breathing exercises is diaphragmatic breathing, also known as belly breathing. This technique focuses on engaging the diaphragm, allowing for deeper, more efficient breaths that can help reduce tension and promote a sense of calm.

Instructions:

- [ ] Sit comfortably in your chair with your feet flat on the floor, spine straight, and hands resting gently on your lap or abdomen.
- [ ] Take a moment to relax your shoulders away from your ears and gently close your eyes or soften your gaze.
- [ ] Begin by slowly exhaling all the air from your lungs through your mouth.
- [ ] Inhale deeply through your nose, directing the breath into your abdomen, and feel your hands rise as your belly expands.
- [ ] Hold the breath for a count of three.
- [ ] Exhale slowly through your mouth, feeling the hands lower as your belly contracts.
- [ ] Repeat this process for several minutes, focusing on the rise and fall of your abdomen and the sensation of full, deep breaths.

Another effective breathing exercise is the 4-7-8 technique, which involves breathing in a specific rhythm to induce relaxation.

Here's how to do it:

- Sit in the same comfortable position, with your back straight and hands resting on your lap.
- Exhale completely through your mouth, making a whoosh sound.

- Close your mouth and inhale quietly through your nose to a mental count of four.
- Hold your breath for a count of seven.
- Exhale completely through your mouth, making a whoosh sound to a count of eight.
- This completes one cycle. Repeat the cycle three more times for a total of four breaths.

The benefits of these guided breathing exercises are numerous, especially for men over 50. Physiologically, they can lower blood pressure, reduce heart rate, and improve circulation, directly combating the effects of stress on the body. Mentally, focusing on the breath helps to clear the mind, improve concentration, and reduce anxiety. Emotionally, the act of deep, mindful breathing can induce a state of calm, helping to alleviate feelings of stress and promote a sense of inner peace.

Additionally, these breathing techniques enhance lung function and respiratory efficiency, which can be particularly beneficial for those dealing with age-related changes in lung capacity. Regular practice can also support improved sleep patterns, making it easier to fall asleep and stay asleep through the night.

Integrating guided breathing exercises into a chair yoga practice offers a holistic approach to health and well-being for men over 50. These exercises provide a simple, yet powerful, tool for managing stress, improving physical health, and fostering a deeper sense of relaxation and peace. By dedicating just a few minutes each day to these practices, individuals can experience significant improvements in their overall quality of life, demonstrating that something as basic as breathing can have profound impacts on our health and happiness.

Seated Meditation Techniques

1. **Choose a Quiet Space**: Select a quiet, comfortable area where interruptions are unlikely. This setting helps in fostering a tranquil environment conducive to meditation.

2. **Proper Seating**: Use a sturdy, armless chair. Sit with your feet flat on the ground, spaced comfortably apart. Ensure your back is straight (to promote good posture) yet relaxed (to avoid tension).

3. **Hand Position**: Place your hands gently on your thighs or knees. Your palms can be facing up or down, depending on what feels most natural and supportive for your meditation practice.

4. **Eyes Closed or Soft Gaze**: Close your eyes to minimize distractions and help internalize your focus. Alternatively, if you prefer, maintain a soft gaze, looking downward a few feet in front of you to reduce eye strain.

5. **Focus on Your Breath**: Begin by taking a few deep breaths, inhaling slowly through your nose and exhaling through your mouth. Then, allow your breath to return to its natural rhythm. Focus your attention on the breath entering and leaving your body. If your mind wanders, gently guide it back to your breath without judgment.

6. **Use of Mantras or Affirmations**: Optionally, you can incorporate a mantra (a word or phrase repeated silently) or affirmations (positive statements) to help maintain

focus and intention during your meditation. Choose something meaningful and calming that resonates with you.

7. **Duration**: Start with a short duration, such as 5 minutes, and gradually increase the time as you become more comfortable with the practice. Consistency is key, so aim to incorporate this practice into your daily routine.

The benefits of incorporating seated meditation into chair yoga for men over 50 are multifaceted. Physically, it can help lower blood pressure, reduce chronic pain, and improve sleep quality. Mentally and emotionally, it enhances stress resilience, boosts mood, increases mindfulness, and cultivates a deeper sense of inner peace. Over time, regular practice of seated meditation can lead to significant improvements in overall quality of life, making it a valuable addition to the wellness routines of men over 50.

The Role of Mindfulness in Stress Reduction

The intricate relationship between mindfulness and stress reduction is profoundly evident in the practice of chair yoga, especially for men over 50. This demographic often faces unique stressors, including health concerns, life transitions, and the challenges of aging. Mindfulness, a core component of yoga, offers a powerful avenue for navigating these stressors with grace and resilience. In chair yoga, mindfulness is not merely an adjunct to physical practice; it is central to transforming the yoga mat into a space of holistic healing and peace.

Mindfulness in the context of chair yoga involves a deliberate, non-judgmental awareness of the present moment. For men over 50, this practice encourages a reconnection with their bodies in a compassionate and accepting manner. It shifts focus from the external pressures and concerns of daily life to the internal experience of breath, movement, and sensation. This shift is crucial for stress reduction, as it moves the practitioner away from stress-inducing patterns of thought and towards a state of calm awareness.

Incorporating mindfulness into chair yoga begins with breath awareness. Men are guided to notice the quality of their breath—its depth, rhythm, and how it feels as it moves through the body. This simple act can significantly lower stress levels by activating the body's parasympathetic nervous system, which promotes relaxation and healing. The mindful breathing practiced in chair yoga serves as a reminder that stress is manageable and that the breath can be a powerful tool in the regulation of emotional states.

The physical poses, or asanas, of chair yoga also serve as a conduit for mindfulness. As men over 50 engage in each pose, they are encouraged to maintain a gentle focus on their bodily sensations and movements. This mindful engagement helps to identify areas of tension and release them, a process that mirrors the release of mental stress. The deliberate, slow pace of chair yoga fosters a meditative state, allowing for deeper introspection and a gradual unwinding of both physical and mental knots.

Mindfulness in chair yoga extends beyond the physical practice, influencing how men over 50 approach life's stressors. Through regular practice, individuals learn to apply the principles of present-moment awareness and non-judgmental acceptance to everyday situations. This ability to stay centered and calm amidst life's ups and downs is perhaps one of the most valuable stress-reduction tools yoga can offer. It encourages a stance of observation rather than reaction, providing a buffer against the stress-inducing stimuli of the external world.

The relaxation and stress reduction benefits of mindfulness in chair yoga are also supported by science. Research has shown that mindfulness can lower cortisol levels, the body's primary stress hormone, and improve markers of well-being. For men over 50, this can translate to better sleep, reduced blood pressure, and an overall enhancement of life quality. The mental clarity and emotional balance fostered by mindfulness can also improve relationships, career satisfaction, and the ability to enjoy life's pleasures.

Chair yoga, with its emphasis on mindful movement and breathing, offers a holistic approach to stress management that is both accessible and effective for men over 50. It acknowledges the complex interplay between mind and body, offering tools that are adaptable to each individual's needs and capacities. By prioritizing mindfulness, chair yoga provides a pathway to not just manage stress but to transform one's relationship with it, leading to a more balanced, peaceful, and fulfilling life.

In conclusion, the role of mindfulness in stress reduction, particularly within the realm of chair yoga for men over 50, cannot be overstated. It equips individuals with the skills to navigate the inevitable stresses of life with grace, resilience, and a sense of inner peace. This practice invites a deeper connection with the self, fostering a sense of well-being that permeates all aspects of life. For men navigating the challenges of midlife and beyond, mindfulness through chair yoga offers a powerful antidote to stress, one that is both nurturing and transformative.

Yoga Sequences for Specific Needs

Yoga for Back Pain Relief

Yoga, with its gentle stretches and focus on alignment, offers significant relief for back pain, a common ailment among men over 50. Chair yoga, in particular, provides a safe, accessible way to enjoy these benefits without the need for getting down on the floor. Through carefully curated sequences, chair yoga can help alleviate back discomfort, improve flexibility, and strengthen the muscles supporting the spine. Here's how men over 50 can use chair yoga for back pain relief, including specific instructions and the benefits of each pose.

Chair Extended Side Angle

Instructions:

- [ ] Sit on the chair sideways with your right side facing the back of the chair.
- [ ] Extend your right leg back, keeping your foot on the floor and your left foot under the knee.

☐ Raise your left arm overhead and reach to the right side. Place your right hand on the back of the chair for support.

☐ Hold for several breaths, then switch sides.

☐ Benefits: Stretches and strengthens the muscles of the sides of the body, improving posture and reducing side back pain.

Seated Spinal Twist

Instructions:

☐ Sit facing forward in your chair.

☐ Place your right hand on the back of the chair and your left hand on your right knee.

☐ Inhale deeply, and on the exhale, gently twist your torso to the right, looking over your right shoulder.

☐ Hold for several breaths, then switch sides.

☐ Benefits: This twist promotes spinal mobility and stretches the back muscles, helping to relieve tension and pain.

Lifestyle and Wellness

Incorporating Yoga Principles into Daily Life

Incorporating yoga concepts into everyday life broadens the advantages of chair yoga beyond the mat, particularly for men over 50. This generation frequently encounters specific problems, such as managing chronic health concerns, adjusting to physical changes, and achieving balance in their home and professional life. Yoga, with its holistic approach to well-being, provides excellent tools for resolving these issues, not just via physical postures but also through its larger philosophical teachings.

One of the fundamental principles of yoga is mindfulness, which promotes living with awareness and intention. For men over 50 who practice chair yoga, mindfulness may convert everyday tasks into moments of intense connection with the present. This might be paying more attention to the body's signals of hunger and fullness, resulting in more mindful eating habits, or noting the breath during stressful periods and applying breath control techniques gained in yoga to develop calm. Mindfulness may also improve relationships since it encourages patience and empathy, allowing for more meaningful interactions with loved ones.

Another important part of yoga is ahimsa, which means nonviolence or harmlessness. Men over 50 can learn to treat themselves with love and compassion by incorporating Ahimsa into their everyday lives, acknowledging and accepting their physical limitations instead of pushing through suffering or discomfort. This soft approach promotes a healthy connection with exercise, with the emphasis on nourishing the body rather than competing or comparing oneself to others.

Satya, or honesty, is another yoga concept with significant consequences for daily life. It promotes honesty with oneself and others, encouraging people to live truly. For men over 50, this may entail identifying their genuine needs and requesting support when necessary, such as asking for assistance with a difficult task or expressing feelings that they may have been trained to hide.

Aparigraha, or non-attachment, stresses the importance of letting go of what no longer benefits us, which is especially essential for this age group. This notion is applicable to tangible goods, bad behaviors, and even obsolete self-perceptions. Men may promote personal growth and resilience by accepting change and letting go of their fear of the unknown.

Saucha, or cleanliness, emphasizes the value of purity in body, mind, and surroundings. For chair yoga practitioners, this might entail having a clutter-free practice area, as well as keeping a clean and tranquil home atmosphere that promotes mental clarity and relaxation. On a personal level, Saucha promotes self-care habits that enhance physical health and hygiene, which contribute to overall well-being.

Brahmacharya, which is generally defined as celibacy, can be construed more broadly as the prudent use of energy. For males over 50, this may entail balancing activity and relaxation, so that energy is not spent on unneeded tensions or diversions. It supports prioritizing activities that feed both the body and the spirit, such as spending time in nature, engaging in creative hobbies, or volunteering, all of which may bring a feeling of purpose and fulfillment.

Finally, Santosha, or contentment, refers to finding satisfaction in the present moment and appreciating what we have. This mindset might fight cultural pressures to constantly seek more or to compare oneself unfavorably with others. For males who practice chair yoga, Santosha promotes gratitude for the body's talents at any age, creating a happy mindset that improves overall quality of life.

Incorporating these yoga concepts into daily life promotes a comprehensive approach to wellbeing, integrating physical health, mental clarity, emotional resilience, and spiritual growth. For men over 50, chair yoga may be the first step toward a more balanced and fulfilled existence, demonstrating that the path to well-being extends well beyond the mat.

Nutrition Tips for Men Over 50

Nutrition is essential for the general health and well-being of men over 50, especially when combined with chair yoga. As the body's natural changes occur with age, a balanced and thoughtful approach to diet becomes increasingly critical in supporting vitality, energy levels, and the benefits of a chair yoga practice.

1. **Balanced Diet**: Men over 50 should focus on eating a range of nutrient-dense meals. This entails including enough of fruits, vegetables, whole grains, lean meats, and healthy fats in their diets. A diversified diet ensures that the body gets the vitamins and minerals it needs to function properly.

2. **Protein Intake:** Protein becomes increasingly important as one ages. Adequate protein consumption preserves muscular mass and strength, which is useful in chair yoga for maintaining stability and balance. Protein-rich foods include lean meats, poultry, fish, lentils, and dairy products.

3. **Hydration**: Maintaining hydration is critical for general health, particularly as men age. Proper hydration promotes joint health and reduces the likelihood of cramping and muscular stiffness during chair yoga practices. Drink plenty of water throughout the day, and try herbal teas or infused water for extra taste.

4. **Healthy Fats**: Consuming healthy fats like avocados, almonds, and olive oil helps improve joint health and decrease inflammation. These fats also improve cognitive function, which is important for mental clarity during chair yoga.

5. **Portion management**: As metabolism slows with age, portion management is critical to maintaining a healthy weight. Chair yoga, along with portion control, can help with weight management and general fitness.

6. **Aware Eating**: Being aware when eating can improve digestion and foster a healthy connection with food. Men over 50 can benefit from eating slowly, savoring each bite, and paying attention to hunger and fullness signs. Mindful eating can improve the mindfulness component of chair yoga, creating inner calm.

7. **Supplements**: While it is important to get nutrients from whole foods, certain men may benefit from supplements, notably vitamin D and calcium, to help with bone health. It is best to contact with a healthcare expert before beginning any supplement program.

8. **Anti-Inflammatory Foods**: Including anti-inflammatory foods such as turmeric, ginger, and berries in your diet will help reduce inflammation in the body. This is especially advantageous

for men who suffer from joint pain, since it allows them to participate in chair yoga more easily.

9. **Fiber-Rich meals**: Fiber-rich meals, such as whole grains and legumes, enhance digestive health and can help with constipation, which may become more frequent as people age. A comfortable digestive system improves the whole chair yoga experience.

10. **Reduce Processed Foods and Sugar**: Limiting processed foods and excessive sugar consumption is critical for maintaining stable energy levels and avoiding chronic health concerns. These dietary changes can improve the efficacy of chair yoga sessions by promoting prolonged energy and attention.

Finally, nutrition suggestions for men over 50 are critical to optimizing the benefits of chair yoga. A balanced and attentive approach to eating not only benefits physical health, but also enhances the mental and emotional components of chair yoga. Men over 50 may make their chair yoga experience more comprehensive and gratifying by fueling their bodies with the correct nutrients and establishing healthy eating habits. This promotes energy, flexibility, and general well being in their later years.

The Importance of Hydration

In the realm of chair yoga for men over 50, where gentle movements and attentive practices are key, one frequently ignored but critical component is water. Staying hydrated is more than simply drinking water; it's an essential component of general health and well-being, particularly as we age.

1. **Maintaining Joint Health**: Men over 50 must prioritize joint health, and water is essential. Adequate hydration keeps the synovial fluid in our joints lubricated, lowering the risk of stiffness and pain. This is especially significant in chair yoga, where mild movements can assist enhance joint mobility and relieve age-related joint pain.

2. **Supporting muscular Function**: Proper muscular function requires enough hydration. Muscles that are properly hydrated are less prone to cramping and injury. Well-hydrated muscles perform better in chair yoga, where preserving strength and flexibility are the major aim, allowing men over 50 to participate more successfully.

3. **Temperature Regulation**: Even though chair yoga is a low-impact exercise, it can cause perspiration. Proper hydration helps to regulate body temperature and prevents overheating during practice. Men over the age of 50 should exercise extra

caution when it comes to temperature management since their bodies may not respond as rapidly to variations in heat.

4. **Cognitive Function:** Staying hydrated is just as important for cognitive function. Dehydration can impair focus, memory, and general mental clarity. Mental clarity is key for getting the most out of chair yoga, which frequently incorporates mindfulness and meditation.

5. **Energy Levels**: Fatigue is a typical problem among males over 50. Dehydration exacerbates fatigue and lethargy. Proper hydration offers the energy required to participate completely in chair yoga sessions, making the practice more pleasurable and successful.

6. **Digestive Health:** Digestive disorders might worsen with age. Hydration is essential for a healthy digestive tract. It prevents constipation and improves the body's capacity to absorb nutrients from meals, ensuring that men over 50 get the most out of their diets.

7. **Heart Health**: Older folks place a high value on heart health. Staying hydrated promotes healthy blood pressure levels. Chair yoga can improve heart health by reducing stress, and when paired with adequate hydration, it provides a comprehensive approach to cardiovascular well-being.

8. **Skin Health**: As we become older, our skin becomes drier and more delicate. Proper hydration promotes skin suppleness while preventing dryness and irritation. This is more than simply appearance; it is about general comfort and well-being.

So, how can men over 50 ensure they stay adequately hydrated in their chair yoga journey?

1. **Drink Water Regularly**: Make a habit of sipping water throughout the day, not just during yoga practice.
2. **Monitor Urine Color**: A pale yellow color indicates good hydration, while dark yellow or amber may suggest dehydration.
3. **Consider Electrolytes**: In some cases, especially after sweating, replenishing electrolytes through sports drinks or electrolyte supplements can be beneficial.
4. **Limit Caffeine and Alcohol**: These can have a diuretic effect and lead to increased fluid loss.
5. **Include Hydrating Foods**: Foods with high water content, like fruits and vegetables, can contribute to hydration.

In conclusion, hydration is a foundational pillar of chair yoga for men over 50. It supports joint health, muscle function, cognitive clarity, energy levels, and overall well-being. By paying attention to their hydration needs, men over 50 can ensure that their chair yoga practice is not only safe but also highly effective in promoting their physical and mental health.

Conclusion

Finally, chair yoga for men over 50 provides a meaningful path toward greater physical and mental health. Throughout this book, we've looked at the numerous aspects of chair yoga, from its mild yet effective postures to its profound effects on flexibility, strength, balance, and relaxation.

Chair yoga offers an inclusive and accessible approach to wellbeing, taking into account the specific requirements and obstacles that men over the age of 50 encounter. It provides a friendly environment in which people can begin their yoga journey without risk of harm. The changes and safety guidelines supplied allow practitioners to tailor the practice to their individual degree of mobility and comfort.

This tutorial has focused on the holistic advantages of chair yoga. It is more than just a physical exercise; it is a lifestyle that encourages awareness, stress reduction, and a stronger connection with one's body. The relaxation and stress-reduction techniques described here extend beyond the mat, providing practitioners with tools to manage life's obstacles more easily.

The strength and flexibility workouts on these pages help men over 50 recover control of their physical health. With persistent practice, individuals can achieve increased muscular tone, joint mobility, and a revitalized sense of vigor. Chair yoga demonstrates that age is not an impediment to obtaining physical fitness and wellness.

Additionally, chair yoga promotes a sense of camaraderie and support. It enables people to connect with others who are going through similar experiences, forming a network of people who inspire and motivate one another. This sense of belonging may be a powerful incentive for achieving improved health.

In conclusion, chair yoga for men over 50 is a practice that transcends age and physical limits. It provides a pathway to better health, more energy, and a more balanced and thoughtful way of life. This guide is only the beginning of a transforming journey, and we hope that individuals who follow it find a new feeling of well-being and resilience that goes well beyond the chair.

15 DAYS WORKOUT TRACKER

DAILY WORKOUT TRACKER

DATE

DAILY MOTIVATION

TODAY'S GOALS

WEATHER

EXECERCISE TYPE

AMOUNT OF WATER

TOTAL :

JOGGING

TOTAL MINUTES

TOTAL STEPS

TODAY'S WORKOUT PLAN

TIME	WORKOUT TYPE

WORKOUT TO GET DONE TODAY

EXERCISE COMPLETED

HEALTHY DIET TRACKER

BREAKFAST	LUNCH
DINNER	SNACKS

NOTES

WORKOUT FOR

DAILY WORKOUT TRACKER

DATE

DAILY MOTIVATION

TODAY'S GOALS

WEATHER

EXECERCISE TYPE

AMOUNT OF WATER

TOTAL :

JOGGING

TOTAL MINUTES

TOTAL STEPS

TODAY'S WORKOUT PLAN

TIME	WORKOUT TYPE

WORKOUT TO GET DONE TODAY

EXERCISE COMPLETED

HEALTHY DIET TRACKER

BREAKFAST	LUNCH
DINNER	SNACKS

NOTES

WORKOUT FOR

DAILY WORKOUT TRACKER

DATE

DAILY MOTIVATION

TODAY'S GOALS

WEATHER

EXECERCISE TYPE

AMOUNT OF WATER

TOTAL :

TODAY'S WORKOUT PLAN

TIME	WORKOUT TYPE

WORKOUT TO GET DONE TODAY

JOGGING

TOTAL MINUTES

TOTAL STEPS

EXERCISE COMPLETED

HEALTHY DIET TRACKER

BREAKFAST	LUNCH
DINNER	SNACKS

NOTES

WORKOUT FOR

DAILY WORKOUT TRACKER

DATE

DAILY MOTIVATION

TODAY'S GOALS

WEATHER

EXECERCISE TYPE

AMOUNT OF WATER

TOTAL :

JOGGING

TOTAL MINUTES

TOTAL STEPS

TODAY'S WORKOUT PLAN

TIME	WORKOUT TYPE

WORKOUT TO GET DONE TODAY

EXERCISE COMPLETED

HEALTHY DIET TRACKER

BREAKFAST	LUNCH
DINNER	SNACKS

NOTES

WORKOUT FOR

DAILY WORKOUT TRACKER

DATE

DAILY MOTIVATION

TODAY'S GOALS

WEATHER

EXECERCISE TYPE

AMOUNT OF WATER

TOTAL :

JOGGING

TOTAL MINUTES

TOTAL STEPS

TODAY'S WORKOUT PLAN

TIME	WORKOUT TYPE

WORKOUT TO GET DONE TODAY

EXERCISE COMPLETED

HEALTHY DIET TRACKER

BREAKFAST	LUNCH
DINNER	SNACKS

NOTES

WORKOUT FOR

DAILY WORKOUT TRACKER

DATE

DAILY MOTIVATION

TODAY'S GOALS

WEATHER

EXECERCISE TYPE

AMOUNT OF WATER

TOTAL :

JOGGING

TOTAL MINUTES

TOTAL STEPS

TODAY'S WORKOUT PLAN

TIME	WORKOUT TYPE

WORKOUT TO GET DONE TODAY

EXERCISE COMPLETED

HEALTHY DIET TRACKER

BREAKFAST	LUNCH
DINNER	SNACKS

NOTES

WORKOUT FOR

DAILY WORKOUT TRACKER

DATE

DAILY MOTIVATION

WEATHER

TODAY'S GOALS

EXECERCISE TYPE

AMOUNT OF WATER

TOTAL :

JOGGING

TOTAL MINUTES

TOTAL STEPS

TODAY'S WORKOUT PLAN

TIME	WORKOUT TYPE

WORKOUT TO GET DONE TODAY

EXERCISE COMPLETED

HEALTHY DIET TRACKER

BREAKFAST	LUNCH
DINNER	SNACKS

NOTES

WORKOUT FOR

DAILY WORKOUT TRACKER

DATE

DAILY MOTIVATION

TODAY'S GOALS

WEATHER

EXECERCISE TYPE

AMOUNT OF WATER

TOTAL :

JOGGING

TOTAL MINUTES

TOTAL STEPS

TODAY'S WORKOUT PLAN

TIME	WORKOUT TYPE

WORKOUT TO GET DONE TODAY

EXERCISE COMPLETED

HEALTHY DIET TRACKER

BREAKFAST	LUNCH
DINNER	SNACKS

NOTES

WORKOUT FOR

DAILY WORKOUT TRACKER

DATE

DAILY MOTIVATION

TODAY'S GOALS

WEATHER

EXECERCISE TYPE

AMOUNT OF WATER

TOTAL :

JOGGING

TOTAL MINUTES

TOTAL STEPS

TODAY'S WORKOUT PLAN

TIME	WORKOUT TYPE

WORKOUT TO GET DONE TODAY

EXERCISE COMPLETED

HEALTHY DIET TRACKER

BREAKFAST	LUNCH
DINNER	SNACKS

NOTES

WORKOUT FOR

DAILY WORKOUT TRACKER

DATE

DAILY MOTIVATION

TODAY'S GOALS

WEATHER

EXECERCISE TYPE

AMOUNT OF WATER

TOTAL :

JOGGING

TOTAL MINUTES

TOTAL STEPS

TODAY'S WORKOUT PLAN

TIME	WORKOUT TYPE

WORKOUT TO GET DONE TODAY

EXERCISE COMPLETED

HEALTHY DIET TRACKER

BREAKFAST	LUNCH
DINNER	SNACKS

NOTES

WORKOUT FOR

DAILY WORKOUT TRACKER

DATE

DAILY MOTIVATION

TODAY'S GOALS

WEATHER

EXECERCISE TYPE

AMOUNT OF WATER

TOTAL :

JOGGING

TOTAL MINUTES

TOTAL STEPS

TODAY'S WORKOUT PLAN

TIME	WORKOUT TYPE

WORKOUT TO GET DONE TODAY

EXERCISE COMPLETED

HEALTHY DIET TRACKER

BREAKFAST	LUNCH
DINNER	SNACKS

NOTES

WORKOUT FOR

DAILY WORKOUT TRACKER

DATE

DAILY MOTIVATION

TODAY'S GOALS

WEATHER

EXECERCISE TYPE

AMOUNT OF WATER

TOTAL :

JOGGING

TOTAL MINUTES

TOTAL STEPS

TODAY'S WORKOUT PLAN

TIME	WORKOUT TYPE

WORKOUT TO GET DONE TODAY

EXERCISE COMPLETED

HEALTHY DIET TRACKER

BREAKFAST	LUNCH
DINNER	SNACKS

NOTES

WORKOUT FOR

DAILY WORKOUT TRACKER

DATE

DAILY MOTIVATION

TODAY'S GOALS

WEATHER

EXECERCISE TYPE

AMOUNT OF WATER

TOTAL :

TODAY'S WORKOUT PLAN

TIME	WORKOUT TYPE

WORKOUT TO GET DONE TODAY

JOGGING

TOTAL MINUTES

TOTAL STEPS

EXERCISE COMPLETED

HEALTHY DIET TRACKER

BREAKFAST	LUNCH
DINNER	SNACKS

NOTES

WORKOUT FOR

DAILY WORKOUT TRACKER

DATE

DAILY MOTIVATION

TODAY'S GOALS

WEATHER

EXECERCISE TYPE

AMOUNT OF WATER

TOTAL :

JOGGING

TOTAL MINUTES

TOTAL STEPS

TODAY'S WORKOUT PLAN

TIME	WORKOUT TYPE

WORKOUT TO GET DONE TODAY

EXERCISE COMPLETED

HEALTHY DIET TRACKER

BREAKFAST	LUNCH
DINNER	SNACKS

NOTES

WORKOUT FOR

DAILY WORKOUT TRACKER

DATE

DAILY MOTIVATION

TODAY'S GOALS

WEATHER

EXECERCISE TYPE

AMOUNT OF WATER

TOTAL :

TODAY'S WORKOUT PLAN

TIME	WORKOUT TYPE

WORKOUT TO GET DONE TODAY

JOGGING

TOTAL MINUTES

TOTAL STEPS

EXERCISE COMPLETED

HEALTHY DIET TRACKER

BREAKFAST	LUNCH
DINNER	SNACKS

NOTES

WORKOUT FOR

Bonus Page

A Group Of Writers Who Take Their Precious Time To Create This Workout Book Have Also Provide You With The Audio Version Of The Book For Free To Enjoy At Your Free Time.

Scan the QR Code Provided below to download it:

www.ingramcontent.com/pod-product-compliance
Lightning Source LLC
Chambersburg PA
CBHW070807260726

48660CB00005B/1755